D0620521

The New MRCPsych Paper I Practice MCQs and EMIs

MUCKAMORE ABBEY HOSPITAL LIBRARY *

The New MRCPsych Paper I Practice MCQs and EMIs

OLIVER WHITE
BMedSci, BM BS, MRCPsych
*Chair, Psychiatric Trainees' Committee,
Royal College of Psychiatrists
Specialist Registrar in Child and Adolescent and Forensic
Psychiatry, Oxford Deanery*

and

CLARE OAKLEY
MB ChB, MRCPsych
*Vice Chair, Psychiatric Trainees' Committee,
Royal College of Psychiatrists
Specialty Registrar, West Midlands Deanery*

Radcliffe Publishing
Oxford • New York

01254040

Radcliffe Publishing Ltd
18 Marcham Road
Abingdon
Oxon OX14 1AA
United Kingdom

www.radcliffe-oxford.com
Electronic catalogue and worldwide online ordering facility.

© 2008 Oliver White and Clare Oakley

Oliver White and Clare Oakley have asserted their right under the Copyright, Designs and Patents Act 1998 to be identified as the authors of this work.

All rights reserved. No part of this publication may be reproduced, stored in a retrieval system or transmitted, in any form or by any means, electronic, mechanical, photocopying, recording or otherwise, without the prior permission of the copyright owner.

British Library Cataloguing in Publication Data

A catalogue record for this book is available from the British Library.

ISBN-13: 978 184619 254 8

Typeset by Pindar NZ (Egan Reid), Auckland, New Zealand
Printed and bound by TJI Digital, Padstow, Cornwall, UK

- 7 APR 2009

Contents

About the authors

Oliver White graduated in 2001 and worked in Nottingham and Sydney, Australia prior to completing his basic psychiatric training on the Mid Trent rotation. He is currently an SpR dual training in Child and Adolescent, and Forensic Psychiatry in the Oxford Deanery. Oliver developed an interest in training issues as an SHO and for the past three years has been a member of the Psychiatric Trainees' Committee of the Royal College of Psychiatrists and is currently Chair of the Committee. He is therefore experienced in the recent changes in psychiatric training, including the development of the new MRCPsych exams.

Clare Oakley graduated from the University of Birmingham in 2003 and undertook her basic psychiatric training in Birmingham, where she is now an ST3. Clare has been a member of the Psychiatric Trainees' Committee of the Royal College of Psychiatrists for the last two years and is currently its Vice Chair. She is involved in developing the curriculum and workplace-based assessments within the Royal College of Psychiatrists and so has an extensive knowledge of the assessment system, including the new MRCPsych exams.

Introduction

Background

The structure of the MRCPsych examination has changed significantly. The exam will no longer consist of two distinct 'Parts' but will consist of three written papers and one clinical exam. This chapter outlines these changes, and further details can be found on the website of the Royal College of Psychiatrists (www.rcpsych.ac.uk). We recommend that candidates check the website carefully before applying to sit the examinations. This book provides 250 practice MCQs and 100 practice EMIs for paper I.

Examination Format

The new written papers will contain 200 questions and will all be three hours long. The papers will include both 'single best answer 1 from 5' style MCQs, and EMIs. The proportion of each type of question in the exam paper may vary but approximately one third of the questions will be EMIs.

There will be a new OSCE-type examination called Clinical Assessment of Skills and Competencies (CASC). It will consist of two parts to be completed in one day. The first part will contain 10 single 'stand alone' stations, each lasting eight minutes (including reading time of one minute). The second part will consist of five pairs of 'linked' stations, which will allow for the assessment of more complex competencies, each lasting 12 minutes (including two minutes reading and preparation time).

Examination Content

The topics tested in each paper are shown in the table below. Broadly speaking, paper I can be considered to be similar to the old style Part 1 written paper; paper II has elements similar to the Part 2 basic sciences paper; paper III is similar to the Part 2 clinical sciences paper with additional critical appraisal and statistics.

Paper I	Paper II	Paper III
History and mental state examination	General principles of psychopharmacology (pharmacokinetics, pharmacodynamics)	Research methods
Cognitive assessment		Evidence-based practice
Neurological examination	Psychotropic drugs	Statistics
Assessment	Adverse reactions	Critical appraisal
Aetiology	Evaluation of treatments	Clinical topics
Diagnosis	Neurosciences (physiology, endocrinology, chemistry, anatomy, pathology)	General Adult
Classification		Liaison
Basic psychopharmacology		Forensic
		Addiction
Basic psychological processes	Genetics	Child and adolescent
Social psychology	Statistics and research (basic)	Psychotherapy
Description and measurement	Epidemiology	Learning disability
Basic psychological treatments	Advanced psychological processes and treatments	Rehabilitation
Human psychological development		Old age psychiatry
Descriptive psychopathology		
Dynamic psychopathology		
Prevention of psychiatric disorder		
History of psychiatry		

Paper I	Paper II	Paper III
Basic ethics and philosophy of psychiatry		
Stigma and culture		

The proportion of questions in each topic in the chapters of this book is based on the indicative breakdown of questions provided by the College.

Techniques for answering questions
MCQs

- Read the question carefully.
- Watch out for double negatives.
- Narrow down the five options by first excluding those that you know are incorrect.
- Phrases which include 'can' 'may' and 'is possible' are often true.
- Phrases which include 'always' 'never' and 'essential' are often false.
- Understand what the following terms mean:
  - Characteristic: you would doubt the diagnosis without this
  - Typical: same as characteristic
  - Pathognomonic: occurs in that disease and no other
  - Specific: same as pathognomonic
  - Recognised: this has been reported
  - Commonly: more than 50%
  - Rare: less than 5%
  - Almost never: 1–2%

EMIs
Each option may be used once, more than once, or not at all.

Each question may have more than one answer (this will be indicated).

It may be helpful to read the question first before reading the answer options.

EMIs take longer than MCQs to answer – make sure you allow enough time.

Recommended reading

Candidates will have their own preferences about textbooks and revision material. We found the following books useful in our preparation for the Membership exams and they cover most of the material required. In the explanatory notes that accompany the answers in this book, there are references to the books below to enable you to read more fully if you have not understood a topic.

General

Fear C. *Essential Revision Notes in Psychiatry for MRCPsych*. Knutsford: PasTest; 2004.

Johnstone E, Cunningham-Owens DG, Lawrie SM *et al.* editors. *Companion to Psychiatric Studies*. 7th ed. London: Churchill Livingstone; 2004.

Levi MI. *Basic Notes in Psychiatry*. 4th ed. Oxford: Radcliffe Publishing; 2005.

Puri BK, Hall AD. *Revision Notes in Psychiatry*. 2nd revised ed. London: Hodder Arnold; 2004.

Psychology

Gross R. *Psychology: the science of mind and behaviour*. 4th revised ed. London: Hodder Arnold; 2001.

Gupta D, Gupta RM, editors. *Psychology for Psychiatrists*. Chichester: John Wiley & Sons; 1999.

Psychopharmacology

Anderson IM, Reid IC, editors. *Fundamentals of Clinical Psychopharmacology*. 3rd revised ed. Abingdon: Taylor & Francis; 2006.

Levi MI. *Basic Notes in Psychopharmacology*. 4th ed. Oxford: Radcliffe Publishing; 2007.

Psychopathology

Casey PR, Kelly B. *Fish's Clinical Psychopathology: signs and symptoms in psychiatry*. 3rd revised ed. London: Gaskell; 2007.

Sims ACP. *Symptoms in the Mind: an introduction to descriptive psychopathology.* 3rd ed. Oxford: Saunders (imprint of Elsevier); 2003.

Assessment and diagnosis

Questions

MCQs

1 Which of the following is not part of the multiaxial classification of DSM-IV?
   a Clinical disorders, and other conditions that may be a focus of clinical attention
   b Global assessment of functioning
   c Level of intelligence
   d Psychosocial and environmental problems
   e General medical conditions

2 Which of the following is a function of the frontal lobe?
   a Abstract conception
   b Shape perception
   c Spatial orientation
   d Verbal memory
   e Language comprehension

3 Which of the following rating scales is completed by an assessor?
   a Hospital Anxiety and Depression (HAD) Scale
   b Visual Analogue Scale for Depression
   c Beck's Depression Inventory (BDI)
   d Hamilton Depression Rating Scale (HAM-D)
   e Clinically Useful Depression Outcome Scale (CUDOS)

4 Which of the following is not routinely included in a mental state examination?

a Observation about the patient's gross movements

b Test of intelligence

c Assessment of insight

d Description of formal thought disorder

e Observation about the patient's rate of speech

5 Which of the following is true regarding magnetic resonance imaging (MRI) of the brain?

a Involves using ionising radiation to study structure

b Shows bony structures clearer than computed tomography (CT) scans

c Takes a shorter period than CT scanning

d Is of little use in the examination of brain stem lesions

e Is generally more expensive than CT scanning

6 Which lesion site causes a lower-left quadrantanopia?

a Right temporal lobe

b Right parietal lobe

c Left temporal lobe

d Left parietal lobe

e Optic chiasm

7 Which of the following is not part of the Mini-Mental State Examination?

a Naming two objects

b Orientation in time

c Writing a sentence

d Recalling date of the First World War

e Orientation in place

8 Which of the following is not a personality disorder as classified in ICD-10?

a Paranoid personality disorder

b Schizoid personality disorder

c Anankastic personality disorder

d Narcissistic personality disorder

e Histrionic personality disorder

9 Which of the following helps differentiate bereavement from a depressive episode?

a Suicidal ideation

b Marked psychomotor retardation

c Symptoms persist for 1 month

d Reduced latency of verbal response

e Anhedonia

10 Which of the following is not classified within the mood (affective) disorders of ICD-10?

a Hypomania

b Mild depressive episode

c Cyclothymia

d Schizoaffective disorder, manic type

e Mania with psychotic symptoms

11 Which of the following is not a characteristic feature of emotionally unstable personality disorder?

a Self-dramatisation

b Impulsivity

c Disturbance in self-image

d Unstable affect

e Unstable relationships

12 Which of the following is not an example of dissociation?

   a Fugue

   b Derealisation

   c Trance

   d Multiple personality

   e Stupor

13 Which of the following is not a cause of optic disc swelling?

   a Hypervitaminosis C

   b Optic neuritis

   c Toxic optic neuropathy

   d Hydrocephalus

   e Chronic hypoxia

14 Which of the following is not suggestive of a cerebellar lesion?

   a Ataxic gait

   b Dysdiadochokinesis

   c Resting tremor

   d Nystagmus

   e Dysarthria

15 Which of the following is correct?

   a The Clinical Interview Scale is not valid for community use.

   b General Health Questionnaire scores fall in physically ill patients.

   c The Hamilton Rating Scale is not valid if used in the physically ill.

   d The Montgomery-Asberg Depression Rating Scale is self-administered.

   e The Beck's Depression Inventory is interviewer based.

16 Which of the following is classified under Organic Disorders in ICD-10?

   a Dissociative motor disorders

   b Atypical bulimia nervosa

c Mental and behavioural disorders due to use of cocaine

d Mild cognitive disorder

e Somatisation disorder

17 The question 'What do you mean when you say you're hearing voices?' is an example of which of the following interview techniques?

a Circular questioning

b Recapitulation

c Confrontation

d Empathy

e Clarification

18 Regarding the Brief Psychiatric Rating Scale (BPRS), which of the following is true?

a It is a self-rating scale.

b It comprises 30 items on a 5-point scale.

c It is particularly suited to patients with major psychiatric illnesses.

d It has a low inter-rater reliability.

e It enables computer-aided diagnosis.

19 Which of the following is not a feature of the somatic syndrome of a depressive episode in ICD-10?

a Decreased energy or increased fatiguability

b Depression worse in the morning

c Marked loss of appetite

d Objective evidence of psychomotor retardation or agitation

e Marked loss of libido

20 Which of the following is a not suggestive of a temporal lobe space-occupying lesion?

a Hallucinations

b Hcadaches

c Seizure

d Hemianopia

e Weight loss

21 Which of the following is not a mental or behavioural disorder specified in ICD-10?

a Nose picking

b Stuttering

c Nail biting

d Thumb sucking

e Hand wringing

22 Which of the following clinical descriptions does not match the neurological sign?

a Calls an apple an orange: semantic paraphrasia

b Shaves only one side of their face: anosagnosia

c Cannot drink through a straw: initiation impairment

d Can describe a face but cannot recognise the person: prosopagnosia

e Has difficulty learning how to use a new cooker: anterograde amnesia

23 Which of the following does not indicate an upper motor neurone lesion?

a Spasticity

b Muscle weakness

c Hyper-reflexia

d Positive Babinski sign

e Fasciculations

24 Which of the following is false in relation to classification?

   a DSM-IV is a hierarchical classification.

   b ICD-10 differentiates categorically between the severity of mental retardation.

   c DSM-IV is operational.

   d Axis III in DSM-IV is concerned with psychosocial issues.

   e The diagnosis of schizophrenia using ICD-10 is reliable.

25 Which of the following is not classified under the ICD-10 F20 Schizophrenia category?

   a Simple schizophrenia

   b Acute schizophrenic-like psychotic disorder

   c Catatonic schizophrenia

   d Hebephrenic schizophrenia

   e Post-schizophrenic depression

26 Which of the following statements is true in relation to post-traumatic stress disorder (PTSD)?

   a Headache is a characteristic symptom.

   b Depression increases vulnerability to PTSD after a traumatic event.

   c PTSD is not associated with emotional blunting.

   d Debriefing immediately after the traumatic event has been shown to decrease the rates of PTSD.

   e PTSD can never be diagnosed more than 6 months after the traumatic event.

27 The statement 'I can see that this is difficult for you to say' is an example of which of the following interview techniques?

   a Open questioning

   b Reflection

   c Empathy

   d Interpretation

   e Sympathy

28 Which of the following fits into Axis III of DSM-IV?
 a Paranoid personality disorder
 b Depression
 c Psychotic disorder due to a medical condition
 d Absence seizures
 e Unemployment

29 Which of the following is inconsistent with a diagnosis of hebephrenic schizophrenia?
 a Hallucinations
 b Affective symptoms
 c Elaborate, systematised delusions
 d Thought disorder
 e Childish behaviour

30 Which of the following instruments consists of standard activities that allow the observation of behaviour?
 a Brief Psychiatric Rating Scale (BPRS)
 b Present State Examination (PSE)
 c Hospital Anxiety and Depression Scale (HADS)
 d Health of the Nation Outcome Scale (HoNOS)
 e Autism Diagnostic Observation Schedule (ADOS)

31 Which of the following diagnoses best matches the description 'Poor functioning and negative symptoms without preceding positive symptoms'?
 a Paranoid schizophrenia
 b Hebephrenic schizophrenia
 c Residual/chronic schizophrenia
 d Simple schizophrenia
 e Undifferentiated schizophrenia

32 Which of the following does not cause ptosis?
 a Left third nerve palsy
 b Myasthenia gravis

c Lambert-Eaton syndrome

d Horner's syndrome

e Left sixth nerve palsy

33 Which of the following is not a routine investigation for a depressed patient?

a Thyroid function tests

b Full blood count

c 24-hour urinary free cortisol

d Serum calcium

e Renal function

34 Which of the following statements about interviewing a depressed patient is false?

a Failure to use direct questions can lead to a failure to establish the severity of a mood disorder.

b Poor assessment of low mood may be due to poor non-verbal skills of the interviewer.

c Commenting on affect can enhance disclosure.

d Commenting on non-verbal behaviour facilitates disclosure.

e Closed questioning should not be used to assess suicidal risk.

35 Which of the following statements about multiple sclerosis (MS) is false?

a Bilateral internuclear ophthalmoplegia is pathognomonic of MS.

b Dissociated sensory loss is a feature.

c Spontaneous remission does not occur.

d It is the most common neurological disease affecting young people.

e Rotational nystagmus is a feature.

36 Which of the following is a test to detect prefrontal lobe pathology?

 a Rey-Osterrieth Test

 b Rivermead Behavioural Memory Test

 c Rorschach Inkblot Test

 d Wisconsin Card Sorting Test

 e Digit Span

37 A 38-year-old woman presents with a 2-month history of reduced energy, low mood, and poor concentration. Investigations show a raised serum calcium level. What is the most likely diagnosis?

 a Hyperthyroidism

 b Cushing's syndrome

 c Hypoparathyroidism

 d Phaeochromocytoma

 e Hyperparathyroidism

38 An absent corneal reflex indicates pathology in which area?

 a Cavernous sinus

 b Jugular foramen

 c Midbrain

 d Cerebellopontine angle

 e Skull base

39 Which of the following is not a standardised diagnostic interview?

 a Present State Examination (PSE)

 b Schedules for Clinical Assessment in Neuropsychiatry (SCAN)

 c Structured Clinical Interview for Diagnosis (SCID)

 d Beck's Depression Inventory (BDI)

 e Composite International Diagnostic Interview (CIDI)

40 Which of the following statements about Alzheimer's dementia is true?

   a There are no known genetic factors.

   b The prevalence of depression is 10%.

   c Personality is more likely to be affected than in vascular dementia.

   d The prevalence is equal among men and women.

   e Early loss of remote memory is a feature.

41 Which of the following is not a test of intelligence?

   a Raven's progressive matrices

   b Wechsler Adult Intelligence Scale-Revised

   c National Adult Reading Test

   d Repertory grid

   e Wechsler Intelligence Scale for Children

42 Which of the following is suggestive of Alzheimer's dementia rather than vascular dementia?

   a History of cerebrovascular disease

   b Fluctuating course

   c Abrupt onset

   d Early nominal dysphasia

   e Focal neurological signs

43 Which of the following is not a personality test?

   a Rorschach inkblot test

   b 16PF

   c MMPI

   d Benton Visual Retention Test

   e Thematic Apperception Test

44 Which of the following is not a feature of Gerstmann's syndrome?

    a Agraphia

    b Right-left disorientation

    c Dyscalculia

    d Constructional apraxia

    e Finger agnosia

45 Which of the following is not a feature of Parkinsonism?

    a Waxy flexibility

    b A resting tremor

    c Cogwheel rigidity

    d Postural abnormalities

    e A festinant gait

46 Which of the following is not characteristic of delirium tremens?

    a Clouding of consciousness

    b Visual hallucinations

    c Auditory illusions

    d Olfactory illusions

    e Lilliputian hallucinations

47 Which of the following neurological signs is not correctly paired with the cause?

    a Cerebellar lesion: dysdiadochokinesis

    b Pseudobulbar palsy: small, spastic tongue

    c Atrophy of caudate nucleus: upper homonymous hemianopia

    d Posterior cerebral artery occlusion: visual hallucinations

    e Left-sided parietal lesion: right-left disorientation

48 Which of the following does not cause the loss of tendon reflexes in the legs?

    a Motor neurone disease

    b Friedreich's ataxia

    c Guillain-Barré syndrome

d Tabes dorsalis

e Charcot-Marie-Tooth syndrome

49 Which of the following would suggest depressive pseudodementia rather than dementia as the diagnosis?

a Conceals memory problem

b Nominal dysphasia

c Ambiguous history

d Frequently answers 'don't know'

e 'Near miss' answers typical

50 The statement 'You mentioned that you have been feeling low for 8 weeks' is an example of which of the following interview techniques?

a Circular questioning

b Recapitulation

c Confrontation

d Empathy

e Clarification

51 Which of the following is not a feature of anankastic personality disorder?

a Rigidity

b Combative and tenacious sense of personal rights

c Excessive pedantry

d Excessive doubt and caution

e Perfectionism that interferes with task completion

52 Which of the following is not a recognised sign or association of anorexia nervosa?

a Increased white cell count

b Osteoporosis

c Hypokalaemia and cardiac arrhythmias

d Increased growth hormone levels

e Reduced gonadotrophins

53 Which of the following is false in relation to puerperal psychosis?

   a It occurs in approximately 1 in 5000 births.

   b It is associated with primigravida.

   c It is more likely to occur in women with a history of bipolar affective disorder.

   d It increases the risk of future psychotic episodes.

   e It is classified under F20 in ICD-10.

54 Which of the following is not supportive of a diagnosis of Lewy body dementia?

   a Fluctuating cognition

   b Visual hallucinations

   c Early deterioration of personality

   d Parkinsonism

   e Neuroleptic sensitivity

55 Which of the following does not commonly occur during manic illness?

   a Grandiose ideas

   b Elation

   c First rank symptoms

   d Irritability

   e Auditory hallucinations

56 Which of the following is not a feature of alcohol dependence?

   a Increased tolerance to alcohol

   b Hallucinosis

   c Reinstatement after abstinence

   d Prominence of drink-seeking behaviour

   e Compulsion to drink

57 Which of the following is not a frontal lobe test?

   a Verbal fluency

   b Stroop effect

   c Thematic Apperception Test

   d Cognitive estimates

   e Trail making test

58 Which of the following is not characteristic of delirium?

   a Clouding of consciousness

   b Elation

   c Visual illusions

   d Disorientation in time

   e Impaired memory

59 Which of the following is not a diagnostic feature of dissocial personality disorder?

   a Callous unconcern for the feelings of others

   b Marked proneness to blame others

   c Incapacity to profit from adverse experience

   d Intense and unstable relationships

   e Very low tolerance to frustration

60 In an acute stress reaction as defined in ICD-10, within what timescale from exposure to the stressor should the onset of symptoms occur?

   a Within 10 minutes

   b Within 30 minutes

   c Within 1 hour

   d Within 1 day

   e Within 1 week

61 Which of the following is not a sexual dysfunction in Chapter V of ICD-10?

   a Organic vaginismus

   b Lack of sexual enjoyment

   c Orgasmic dysfunction

   d Premature ejaculation

   e Non-organic dyspareunia

62 Which of the following is not an autonomic symptom of anxiety?

a Sweating

b Shortness of breath

c Trembling

d Dry mouth

e Palpitations

63 Which of the following is not a catatonic behaviour?

a Stupor

b Posturing

c Rigidity

d Command automatism

e Apathy

64 Which of the following cranial nerves is incorrectly named?

a 5th – Trigeminal

b 9th – Glossopharyngeal

c 10th – Accessory

d 7th – Facial

e 4th – Abducens

65 Which of the following is not part of the Edwards and Gross Alcohol Dependence Syndrome?

a Narrowing of drinking repertoire

b Tolerance

c Withdrawal

d Binge drinking

e Rapid reinstatement

66 Which of the following is not a clinical feature of bulimia nervosa?

a Craving of food

b Endocrine imbalance

c Alternating periods of starvation

d Self-perception of being too fat

e Self-induced purging

67 Which of the following is not a feature of schizoid personality disorder?

a Odd beliefs or magical thinking

b Excessive preoccupation with fantasy

c Eccentricity

d Emotional detachment

e Withdrawal from close relationships

68 Which of the following statements about mania is false?

a Lack of insight is a characteristic feature.

b Clouding of consciousness is compatible with the diagnosis.

c Inappropriate behaviour is compatible with the diagnosis.

d Irritability is a characteristic feature.

e Stupor is compatible with the diagnosis.

EMIs

1 Diagnosis of anxiety disorders:

a Post-traumatic stress disorder

b Social phobia

c Acute stress reaction

d Generalised anxiety disorder

e Adjustment reaction

f Phobic disorder

g Panic disorder

h Agoraphobia

i Mixed anxiety and depressive disorder

Select the most appropriate diagnosis for the following individuals:

1 A 54-year-old woman observed her husband having a myocardial infarction at home. When her husband was recovering on the coronary care unit she was noticed to be trembling, sweating and very anxious. When approached by staff she became very agitated and abusive.

2 A 36-year-old bank clerk was held at gunpoint during an armed robbery. She does not return to work and avoids going to other banks. She complains of flashbacks and feeling anxious all the time.

3 A 29-year-old man complains of chest pains, headaches, dizziness and anxiety symptoms for which no physical cause is found. He feels fearful and on edge all the time.

4 A 45-year-old woman has been frightened to go out of her house and fears she is going to die before she has to leave the house to attend an appointment. She has recently started to abuse alcohol.

2 Diagnosis:
   a Bipolar affective disorder
   b Schizophrenia
   c Depressive episode
   d Generalised anxiety disorder
   e Manic episode
   f Dementia
   g Panic disorder
   h Emotionally unstable personality disorder

Select the most appropriate diagnosis for the following individuals:

1 A 66-year-old man has been feeling sad for 3 months. He doesn't want to do anything and has no motivation.

2 A 21-year-old complains of low mood for 4 years and has a history of multiple episodes of self-harm. She was sexually abused as a teenager.

3 A 19-year-old student presents with persecutory ideas, perplexity and lack of concentration. His academic performance has deteriorated.

3 Symptomatology:

a She feels very tired with no energy.

b Her beliefs are encapsulated.

c When she sees a blue car passing she realises she is being chased by the IRA.

d She believes she has always been a failure and will never achieve anything.

e She has begun to have difficulty with her hearing.

f She believes she is a famous pop singer.

g She believes that her bowels are rotting away.

h She has functioned well throughout her life and maintained a good employment record.

i She has had previous episodes of mood disorder.

j She believes thoughts are put into her mind that are not her own.

k When she eats she hears a voice saying 'look at her, she's eating'.

Which of the symptoms above would be most likely to be found in the following situations?

1 A 68-year-old woman accuses her neighbours of trying to harm her and steal her belongings. She clearly hears them talking about her through the walls of the house. (3 answers)

2   A 45-year-old woman presents feeling low in mood with weight loss and suicidal ideation. (4 answers)

3   A 27-year-old woman says she is being controlled by a satellite which makes her look sad. (3 answers)

4   A 33-year-old woman presents feeling elated and having difficulty sleeping. (2 answers)

4   Diagnosis of dementia:
   a   Sudden onset
   b   Motor features of Parkinson's disease
   c   Personality change
   d   Overeating
   e   Visual hallucinations
   f   Gradual onset
   g   Disinhibition
   h   Myoclonus
   i   Autoscopy
   j   Step-wise deterioration

Select 2 features from the above that are characteristic of:

1   Lewy body dementia

2   Frontal lobe dementia

3   Vascular dementia

5   Investigations:
   a   Full blood count
   b   Thyroid function tests
   c   Blood gases
   d   Liver function tests
   e   Urine drug screen
   f   Discussion with informant

g Mini-Mental State Examination

h Paracetamol and salicylate levels

i Fasting glucose

Select 3 of the above investigations for these situations:

1 A 77-year-old woman is brought to hospital. She is withdrawn, not eating, not taking care of herself and has been experiencing suicidal thoughts for the last 6 months. Her problems have worsened since the death of her husband 6 weeks ago. She has been taking antihypertensives for many years.

2 A 48-year-old man was brought to A+E after he tried to hang himself. He has a history of alcohol and drug problems. He is found to be depressed, more subjectively than objectively.

6 Disorders of memory:

a Transient global amnesia

b Non-organic amnesic syndrome

c Jamais vu

d Retrograde amnesia

e Confabulation

f Déjà vu

g Anterograde amnesia

h Amnesic syndrome

i Dissociative amnesia

Which of the above memory disorders are described below?

1 A falsification of memory occurring in clear consciousness in association with amnesia

2 Amnesia for events occurring after a head injury

3 An experience which the patient knows he has experienced before is not associated with the appropriate feeling of familiarity

4 Memory loss is usually centred on traumatic events and is usually partial and selective

Answers

MCQs

1 c

There are five axes in the DSM-IV diagnostic system – the four other options plus Personality Disorders and Mental Retardation. (Puri, Hall, p. 311)

2 a

For a list of frontal lobe functions *see* Puri, Hall, pp. 60–1.

3 d

The rest are self-rated.

4 b

Estimation of intelligence may be made but formal testing is not completed.

5 e

MRI is more expensive than CT scanning.

6 b

A temporal lobe lesion would cause a superior quadrantanopia.

7 d

8 d

This is classified in DSM-IV but not ICD-10.

9 b

This is suggestive of a depressive episode. (Puri, Hall, p. 83)

10 d

This is classified under schizophrenia, schizotypal and delusional disorders.

11 a

This is a feature of histrionic personality disorder.

12 b

Dissociative stupor can be stress related. (Puri, Hall, p. 419)

13 a

Hypervitaminosis A is a cause.

14 c

There is an intention tremor in cerebellar lesions.

15 c

Physical illness is likely to confound the results.

16 d

Mild cognitive disorder is classified under ICD-10 (code F06.7). Mental and behavioural disorders caused by substances are a separate category under ICD-10.

17 e

18 c

It is particularly suited to patients with major psychiatric illnesses and is commonly used to evaluate change in symptoms over time for schizophrenia.

19 a

This is one of the three core features of depression but is not part of the somatic syndrome.

20 d

Hemianopia is a localising sign of the occipital lobe.

21 e

All the other options are classified with behavioural and emotional disorders with onset usually occurring in childhood and adolescence.

22 c

Being unable to drink through a straw would occur in buccofacial apraxia.

23 e

This is a sign of a lower motor neurone lesion.

24 d

Axis III is concerned with general medical conditions. (Puri, Hall, p. 311)

25 b

This is classified under Acute and transient psychotic disorders (F23).

26 b

PTSD can be diagnosed if onset occurs after 6 months, but should be clearly specified according to ICD-10.

27 c

Empathy is the capacity to think and feel into the inner life of another person.

28 d

Axis III defines medical disorders.

29 c

Delusions are common in hebephrenic schizophrenia but should not be elaborate and should not dominate the clinical picture.

30 e

31 d

As described in ICD-10.

32 e

Cranial nerve VI lesions cause squint and nystagmus.

33 c

24-hour urinary free cortisol is the screening test for Cushing's syndrome and is not done routinely.

34 e

The assessment of suicidal risk needs to include closed questions to ensure thoroughness.

35 c

36 d

37 e

38 d

A cerebellopontine angle lesion also presents with sensorineural deafness.

39 d

BDI is self-administered.

40 c

41 d

Repertory grid assesses personality. (Puri, Hall, p. 39)

42 d

43 d

The Benton Visual Retention Test is a memory test. (Puri, Hall, pp. 99–100)

44 d

Constructional apraxia results from a non-dominant occipital lobe lesion. (Puri, Hall, p. 61)

45 a

(Puri, Hall, p. 149)

46 d

(Fear, p. 482)

47 c

Atrophy of the caudate nucleus occurs in Huntingdon's disease resulting in choreiform movements.

48 a

Motor neurone disease affects upper and lower motor neurones and so reflexes are increased in the presence of muscle wasting and fasciculation.

49 d

50 b

51 b

A tenacious sense of personal rights occurs in paranoid personality disorder.

52 a

The white cell count is low.

53 e

It is poorly defined in ICD-10 but can be classified under F53.

54 c

This is more consistent with frontotemporal dementia.

55 c

Auditory hallucinations occur in 30–40%. First rank symptoms of schizophrenia occur in 10% (therefore not 'common').

56 b

Hallucinosis may occur in chronic excessive alcohol intake but is not part of the dependence syndrome.

57 c

The Thematic Apperception Test is a projective personality test. (Puri, Hall, p. 100)

58 b

The mood is more usually anxious or depressed.

59 d

This is a feature of emotionally unstable personality disorder. In dissocial personality disorder there is an incapacity to maintain enduring relationships.

60 c

61 a

Non-organic vaginismus is a Chapter V ICD-10 disorder but organic causes of sexual dysfunction are specifically excluded.

62 b

Shortness of breath as an anxiety symptom is grouped under those involving the chest and abdomen rather than under the autonomic arousal symptoms (*see* ICD-10 criteria for panic disorder/general anxiety disorder).

63 e

Apathy is a negative symptom of schizophrenia.

64 c

The accessory nerve is the 11th cranial nerve.

65 d

Binge drinking is not a feature of alcohol dependence but causes physical and social harm.

66 b

Although weight loss frequently occurs in bulimia nervosa, it is rarely to the extent of causing an endocrine imbalance.

67 a

Odd beliefs or magical thinking are a feature of schizotypal disorder.

68 b

EMIs

1 1 c

   2 a

   3 d

   4 h

2 1 c

   2 h

   3 b

3 1 b, e, h

2 a, d, g, i

3 c, j, k

4 f, i

4 1 b, e

2 c, g

3 a, j

5 1 b, f, g

2 c, d, e

6 1 e

2 g

3 c

4 i

Basic psychopharmacology

Questions

MCQs

1 Which of the following is not an acute dystonia?
   a Oculogyric crisis
   b Akathisia
   c Torticollis
   d Tongue protrusion
   e Facial grimacing

2 Which of the following factors does not affect drug absorption?
   a Gastric pH
   b Glomerular filtration rate (GFR)
   c Gastric emptying
   d Intestinal microflora
   e Intestinal motility

3 Which of the following is not a feature of autonomic dysfunction?
   a Constipation
   b Tachycardia
   c Pallor
   d Urinary incontinence
   e Sweating

4   Regarding oral drug administration, which of the following is true?

   a   Drugs are absorbed primarily by active transport.

   b   Drugs are absorbed mainly in the stomach.

   c   Drugs are absorbed better in ionised form.

   d   Drugs are absorbed less readily in the presence of food.

   e   Drugs are absorbed more quickly than when given by intravenous injection.

5   Regarding opiates, which of the following is false?

   a   Opiate receptors are found in the thalamus.

   b   Opiates decrease respiratory rate.

   c   Opiates decrease the sensitivity of the respiratory centre to carbon dioxide.

   d   Opiates can be used as an antiemetic.

   e   Opiates can cause dependency.

6   Which of the following is not true in relation to drug absorption and distribution?

   a   Most psychotropic drugs are lipid soluble.

   b   Parenteral administration of drugs avoids the first pass effect.

   c   The first pass effect is the pre-systemic metabolism of orally administered drugs.

   d   Psychotropic drugs in the plasma are largely present in the unbound form.

   e   Plasma protein binding reduces drug distribution.

7   Which of the following is not a feature of neuroleptic malignant syndrome?

   a   Hyperthermia

   b   Altered level of consciousness

   c   Flaccid muscles

   d   Tachycardia

   e   Increased level of creatinine phosphokinase

8 Which of the following is true in relation to the blood brain barrier?

   a Drugs with high lipid partition coefficients have increased permeability through the blood brain barrier.

   b Dopamine passes through the blood brain barrier.

   c Drugs that are in highly ionised form have increased permeability through the blood brain barrier.

   d Drugs with high plasma protein binding have increased permeability through the blood brain barrier.

   e Intranasal sprays bypass the blood brain barrier.

9 Which of the following is false in relation to metabolism and elimination?

   a Metabolism of psychotropic drugs involves converting them into more water-soluble forms.

   b Most psychotropic drugs follow zero order kinetics.

   c A proportion of drug is partly excreted in the bile and is partly reabsorbed from the intestine.

   d Psychotropic drugs are metabolised mainly by the liver.

   e In first order kinetics the rate of drug elimination is proportional to its plasma concentration.

10 Which of the following is false in relation to psychopharmacology in the elderly?

   a The renal blood flow is decreased.

   b The pharmacokinetics are affected by reduced total body water.

   c There is decreased hepatic enzyme activity.

   d The receptor sensitivity is decreased.

   e They should be started on low doses of psychotropic drugs.

11 Which of the following is not an SSRI?

   a Sertraline

   b Fluvoxamine

   c Citalopram

   d Clomipramine

   e Paroxetine

12 Which of the following is not a feature of benzodiazepine withdrawal?

   a Sedation

   b Tremor

   c Muscle twitching

   d Anxiety

   e Seizures

13 Which of the following is not a recognised side effect of tricyclic antidepressants?

   a Dry mouth

   b Sexual dysfunction

   c Cardiac arrhythmia

   d Postural hypotension

   e Weight loss

14 Which of the following is false in relation to psychopharmacology in pregnancy?

   a Gastric motility is decreased.

   b The permeability of the blood brain barrier is greater in a foetus than in an adult.

   c SSRIs are generally considered safe in pregnancy.

   d Hepatic metabolism is increased.

   e The GFR is decreased.

15 Which of the following antipsychotics is not available as a depot formulation?

a Haloperidol

b Risperidone

c Zuclopenthixol

d Flupenthixol

e Trifluoperazine

16 Which of the following is not an anticholinergic?

a Nifedipine

b Benzhexol

c Procyclidine

d Orphenadrine

e Benztropine

17 Which of the following is not a treatment for dementia?

a Rivastigmine

b Galantamine

c Memantine

d Donepezil

e Tetrabenazine

18 Which of the following is not correct regarding classification of antipsychotics?

a Trifluoperazine: phenothiazine

b Chlorpromazine: thioxanthine

c Risperidone: benzisoxazole

d Amisulpiride: substituted benzamide

e Clozapine: dibenzodiazepine

EMIs

1   Extra-pyramidal side effects of antipsychotics:
  a Muscle spasm
  b Bradykinesia
  c Develop after long-term treatment
  d Constantly pacing up and down
  e Develop days to weeks after starting treatment
  f Lip smacking
  g Torticollis
  h Can develop within hours of starting medication
  i Tongue protrusion
  j Tremor

Which of the above side effects are features of the following?

  1 Acute dystonia (2 answers)

  2 Parkinsonism (3 answers)

  3 Akathisia (2 answers)

  4 Tardive dyskinesia (3 answers)

2   Mood stabilisers:
  a Lithium
  b Carbamazepine
  c Sodium valproate
  d Lamotrigine
  e Topiramate
  f Olanzapine
  g Quetiapine

The following statements refer to which of the above mood stabilisers?

1　Potentiates the effects of warfarin

2　Causes weight loss

3　Is associated with rashes (2 answers)

4　Was first used in psychiatric patients by John Cade in the 1950s

Answers

MCQs

1 b

Akathisia is not an acute dystonia. (Anderson, Reid, p. 47)

2 b

(Puri, Hall, p. 244)

3 a

(Puri, Hall, p. 261)

4 d

The presence of food delays gastric emptying and therefore delays transit to the small intestine where the majority of drugs are absorbed. (Puri, Hall, p. 244)

5 d

Opiates commonly cause nausea.

6 d

7 c

Increased tone is a feature. (Puri, Hall, p. 261)

8 a

(Puri, Hall, p. 247)

9 b

Most psychotropic drugs follow first order kinetics.

10 d

11 d

Clomipramine is a tricyclic antidepressant.

12 a

Insomnia is a feature.

13 e

Tricyclic antidepressants commonly cause weight gain.

14 e

15 e

16 a

Nifedipine is a calcium-channel blocker.

17 e

Tetrabenazine is used in Huntington's chorea (BNF).

18 b

Chlorpromazine is a phenothiazine.

EMIs

1 1 a, h

   2 b, e, j

   3 d, e

   4 c, f, i

2 1 c

   2 e

   3 b, d

   4 a

Basic psychology

Questions

MCQs

1   Which of the following is not a Gestalt principle?
    a   Similarity
    b   Proximity
    c   Closure
    d   Constancy
    e   Continuity

2   Which of the following is not related to classical conditioning?
    a   Positive reinforcement
    b   Unconditioned stimulus
    c   Conditioned response
    d   Extinction
    e   Reciprocal inhibition

3   Which of the following is the highest level in Maslow's hierarchy of needs?
    a   Self-esteem
    b   Survival
    c   Self-actualisation
    d   Cognitive activity
    e   Safety

4 Which of the following is not true about language development in children?

  a Rate of language development is linked to intelligence.

  b Skinner proposed that acquisition of language is acquisition of a rule system and code.

  c Bruner saw the basis of grammar in preverbal social exchange between mother and child.

  d Chomsky demonstrated that children can invent their own grammar rules.

  e Children become proficient in language because of what they hear others say.

5 Which of the following is true regarding attachment?

  a Attachment to the father cannot be as strong as to the mother.

  b Attachment is better in children adopted after 2 months of age.

  c A maternal substitute interferes with attachment.

  d By the end of the first year of life a close attachment to a mother figure should have been established.

  e A child who is not adopted until 2 months of age has an increased risk of emotional disorders.

6 Which of the following is the type of memory that contains specific events in your life?

  a Implicit memory

  b Primary memory

  c Episodic memory

  d Semantic memory

  e Declarative memory

7 Which of the following is not one of the stages in psychosexual development as described by Freud?

  a Oral stage

  b Anal stage

  c Phallic stage

d Penis envy stage

e Latent stage

8 Which of the following leads to an increase in cognitive dissonance?

a Denigrating what we cannot achieve

b When behaviour is altered

c When cognitions are ignored

d When there is pressure to comply

e When cognitions are added

9 Which of the following schedules of reinforcement occurs in gambling?

a Continuous reinforcement

b Fixed interval reinforcement

c Fixed ratio reinforcement

d Variable interval reinforcement

e Variable ratio reinforcement

10 Which of the following is false in relation to attitude change?

a Low self-esteem and intelligence of the recipient increases the likelihood that complex communications will be persuasive.

b Message repetition can be a persuasive influence.

c Interactive personal discussions are more persuasive than mass media communication.

d Implicit messages are more persuasive for the more intelligent recipient.

e Attractive people are more persuasive communicators.

11 Regarding language development, which of the following is incorrect?

   a By 3–4 months, babbling occurs.

   b By 18 months, a 20–50 word vocabulary is expressed in single-word utterances.

   c By 8 months, the phrases 'mama' and 'dada' are used.

   d By 3 years, a child can usually understand a request containing 3 parts.

   e By 2 years, 2 or 3 word utterances are strung together.

12 Which of the following is not a test of memory?

   a Rey-Osterrieth Test

   b Boston Naming Test

   c WMS-R

   d Benton Visual Retention Test

   e Paired associate learning tests

13 Which of the following is the most life-changing according to the Holmes-Rahe life events scale?

   a Death of a spouse

   b Retirement

   c Divorce

   d Going to prison

   e Pregnancy

14 Which of the following statements about the process of learning of new behaviour is true?

   a Habituation is a complex form of learning.

   b Conditioned stimulus is usually of biological significance.

   c In classical conditioning subjects are passive.

   d The main effect of operant conditioning is to increase the number of different stimuli to elicit a given response.

   e In classical conditioning new behaviour can be learnt.

15 Which of the following is not characteristic of models from which observational learning takes place most effectively?

   a High status

   b High competence

   c High social power

   d High speed while talking

   e High attractiveness

16 Which of the following is true of Thomas and Chess's New York Longitudinal Study (NYLS) of temperament?

   a It was based on the assumption that temperament is largely genetically determined.

   b It used the Child Behavioural Checklist to formulate the dimensions of temperament.

   c It recruited the sample from a homogeneous middle-class group of parents.

   d Activity levels accounted for the greatest variation between children.

   e Slow-to-warm-up babies were predisposed to developing later behaviour disorders.

17 In associative learning, the optimum delay between the unconscious stimulus and the conditioned stimulus is:

   a 0.1 seconds

   b 0.5 seconds

   c 1 second

   d 2 seconds

   e 5 seconds

18 Which of the following is incorrect regarding Kohlberg's theories of moral development?

a There are three levels of morality.

b Stages are parallel to those of Piaget's stages of cognitive development.

c Often children do not progress through stages sequentially.

d The highest stages are very rarely achieved and cannot be regarded as normal.

e Only 50% of the population reach the highest level of moral development.

19 Which of the following is true regarding operant conditioning?

a Discrimination can occur.

b Extinction cannot occur.

c Punishment is a type of negative reinforcement.

d In partial reinforcement, all of the conditioned responses are partially reinforced.

e A negative reinforcer reduces the probability of occurrence of an operant behaviour.

20 Which of the following factors is inversely correlated with intelligence?

a Birth order

b Age

c Parental IQ

d Marital status

e Height

21 In Ainsworth's 'Strange Situation' original experiment (1978), what percentage of one year olds were securely attached?

a 20%

b 35%

c 55%

d 70%

e 85%

22 Which of the following behaviours does not indicate separation anxiety?

a Increased aggressive behaviour

b Developmental retardation

c Psychosomatic reactions

d Clinging behaviour

e Detachment

23 Which of the following are not theories of forgetting?

a Trace decay

b Interference

c Retrograde amnesia

d Cue-dependent forgetting

e Repression

24 Which of the following techniques cannot be used to improve memory?

a Shaping

b Chunking

c Mnemonic techniques

d Mood-dependent techniques

e Rehearsal

25 Which of the following is not a form of long-term memory?

a Episodic

b Semantic

c Autobiographical

d Implicit

e Working memory

26 Which of the following is true regarding Piaget's stages of development?

   a Children in the formal operational stage can show abstract thinking.

   b The pre-operational stage is between 6 and 18 months of age.

   c Conservation of mass can be readily demonstrated in the pre-operational stage.

   d Accommodation means relating new experiences to existing schemas.

   e The egocentrism concept is based on the fact that the child is only concerned about their own needs.

27 Which of the following is not one of the 'big five' personality traits?

   a Openness

   b Conscientiousness

   c Neuroticism

   d Agreeableness

   e Psychoticism

28 Regarding emotions, which of the following is true?

   a Basic emotions are those that require lesser cognitive processing.

   b The James-Lange theory postulates that emotional experience occurs in response to the detection of physiological state.

   c The Canon-Bard theory states that the experience of emotion is dependent on feedback of visceral sources.

   d The Canon-Bard theory argues that emotional experience is a direct result of activation of the autonomic nervous system.

   e The Schachter-Singer theory does not involve cognitive labelling.

29 Which of the following is false in relation to bystander intervention?

   a Impulsive helping is more common in an emergency.

   b Males are more likely to intervene than females.

   c Females are more empathic than males.

   d Chivalry is more common in males.

   e Personality differences in relation to intervention have been consistently reported.

30 Which of the following is not true regarding neonatal social development?

   a Smiling becomes discriminatory after 3 months.

   b Infants show a preference for the mother's face over other face-type configurations after a few days.

   c Infants with wide cheeks, short faces and large wide-set eyes have been shown to be the most appealing to adults.

   d The neonate has an internal representation of self.

   e The neonate is not distressed at separation from the mother.

31 Which of the following is not a criticism of the theory of human aggression proposed by Lorenz?

   a Early man was a hunter-gatherer rather than a warrior.

   b Other primates also kill each other.

   c Aggression in animals is generally considered to be reactive rather than spontaneous.

   d It is based on the study of non-primates.

   e It does not account for learning.

32 Which of the following is false regarding short term memory?

   a It has a capacity of 7+2 units.

   b Its capacity can be expanded by chunking.

   c Rehearsal is easily disrupted.

   d Encoding is primarily echoic.

   e It has a duration of 0.5 seconds.

33 Which of the following is false with regard to gender?

  a Gender constancy is developed during adolescence.

  b Gender identity is established by the age of 4 years.

  c Homosexuals have normal gender identity.

  d Transsexuals have abnormal gender identity.

  e Gender stability is established by the age of 6 years.

34 Which of the following is true with regard to arousal?

  a The response to a stimulus is linear.

  b The Yerkes-Dodson law is U-shaped.

  c Performance is maximal with minimal arousal.

  d Arousal can be measured using galvanic skin response.

  e Maximal arousal is desirable for optimum performance.

35 Which of the following is false with regard to aggression?

  a Vicarious catharsis is common.

  b It is more likely in the presence of a weapon.

  c Vicarious learning is stressed in social learning theory.

  d It is an innate response according to the frustration-aggression hypothesis.

  e Observation of television violence increases aggression in children.

36 Which of the following is true with regard to long-term memory?

  a It has a limited capacity.

  b It accounts for the primacy effect.

  c It is susceptible to state-dependent learning.

  d It accounts for the recency effect.

  e Encoding is echoic.

37 Which of the following is not associated with classical conditioning?

a Stimulus preparedness

b Negative reinforcement

c Incubation

d Extinction

e Higher-order conditioning

38 Which of the following is false in relation to Freud?

a Anxiety results from conflict between the ego and the id.

b Id anxiety is the fear of giving in to primitive impulses.

c Sibling rivalry is seen in the phallic stage.

d Sexual conflict occurs in the latency stage.

e The primary drive is always an unconscious process.

39 Which of the following is true regarding operant conditioning?

a Shaping refers to the procedure of positively reinforcing successive approximations of a goal behaviour.

b Negative reinforcement and punishment are identical processes.

c Reinforcement can occur before the behaviour.

d Punishment is most effective when it starts at low intensity and builds up over repeated trials.

e Behaviours which are intermittently reinforced are both quicker to learn and more resistant to extinction.

40 Which of the following is false with regard to learned helplessness?

a The punishment is contingent on the action.

b It was first described by Seligman.

c It results from a failure to escape from stressful situations.

d It was demonstrated in animal experiments.

e It can be used to describe the behaviour of people who are depressed.

41 Which of the following is false regarding classical conditioning?

    a Extinction is the disappearance of a conditioned response on discontinuation of the unconditioned stimulus.

    b It is most efficient when the time interval between conditioned and unconditioned stimulus is 0.5 seconds.

    c Stimulus generalisation refers to the ability of the same stimulus to evoke subtly differing conditioned responses.

    d A previously conditioned stimulus becoming an unconditioned stimulus is termed higher-order learning.

    e It can only occur if there is already some link between the stimulus and response.

42 Which of the following is not associated with operant conditioning?

    a Punishment

    b Positive reinforcement

    c Variable ratio reinforcement

    d Higher-order conditioning

    e Negative reinforcement

43 Regarding measurement scales in psychology, which of the following is false?

    a The Likert scale is a five-point scale.

    b The semantic differential scale has a low test-retest reliability but is easy to use.

    c The Likert scale can lead to differing response patterns resulting in the same mean score.

    d The Thurstone scale is a dichotomous scale indicating agreement or disagreement with presented statements.

    e The semantic differential scale is a visual analogue scale.

44 Which of the following is not associated with delayed language development?

    a Being male

    b Being a twin

    c Larger family size

d Bilingual home

e Prolonged second stage of labour

45 Which of the following is true in relation to the paranoid-schizoid position?

a Repression is used as a defence mechanism.

b It is associated with delusions.

c Projective identification is used as a defence mechanism.

d It predisposes to personality disorders.

e It causes developmental delay.

46 Which of the following statements is true about the development of antisocial behaviour?

a Twin and adoption studies have reported a strong genetic influence in juvenile delinquency.

b There is research evidence to show that antisocial behaviour is more closely related to social class than to environmental influence.

c Recent studies have shown a direct relationship between delinquency and family size.

d Family discord is more important than family breakdown as a predictor of future delinquency.

e Multiple regression techniques are better predictors of delinquency than linear methods.

47 Which of the following is not an innate fear?

a Noise

b Height

c Pain

d Falling

e Sudden motion

48 Regarding Piaget's stages of cognitive development, which of the following is incorrect?

a External reality is not distinct from self in the sensorimotor stage.

b Objective conception is acquired early.

c Egocentricity characterises the preoperational stage.

d The boundary between concrete and formal operational stages is not clear.

e Hypothesising is not achieved until the age of 12.

49 Which of the following is incorrect regarding imprinting?

a Imprinting is reversible.

b Imprinting is limited to a very brief period.

c Imprinting is limited to mammals.

d When abnormal, it is a reason why animals reared in captivity have difficulty mating.

e Imprinting occurs in humans.

50 Which of the following is not an attachment style as defined in the Adult Attachment Interview (AAI)?

a Anxious-ambivalent

b Dismissing

c Unresolved/Disorganised

d Preoccupied/Entangled

e Secure/Autonomous

51 Which of the following is not a stage of dying as defined by Kübler-Ross?

a Anger

b Guilt

c Acceptance

d Bargaining

e Depression

52 Which of the following was described by Margaret Mahler?

a Genital stage

b Social contact stage

c Autistic phase

d Concrete operational phase

e Good boy – nice girl orientation

53 By what age should a child be able to stack 4 to 6 blocks on top of each other?

a 4–6 months

b 12 months

c 18 months

d 24 months

e 36 months

54 By what age should a child be able to point to one named body part?

a 12 months

b 18 months

c 24 months

d 30 months

e 36 months

EMIs

1 Memory:
   a Recency
   b Encoding
   c Procedural memory
   d Declarative episodic memory
   e Sensory store
   f Recall
   g Declarative semantic memory
   h Working memory
   i Retroactive inhibition
   j Primacy
   k Retrieval

Which aspect of memory is described below?

   1 Influence recall in the short-term memory (2 answers)

   2 Can be assessed by digit span

   3 Forgetting may be due to a failure of this

   4 Also known as biographical memory

2 Conditioning:
   a Positive reinforcement
   b Chaining
   c Modelling
   d Learned helplessness
   e Covert sensitisation
   f Negative reinforcement
   g Punishment
   h Shaping

Match the terms above with the descriptions below:

1 A speeding motorist is stopped by the police and given a ticket.

2 A child hits his brother after watching a violent television programme.

3 A person with learning disability is first taught the components of a more complex desired behaviour.

4 A woman complains of feeling sad and unmotivated, as she feels that nothing she does changes the many stressors and difficulties in her life.

3 Operant conditioning:
   a Time out
   b Fixed ratio reinforcement
   c Punishment
   d Negative reinforcement
   e Shaping
   f Positive reinforcement
   g Fixed interval reinforcement
   h Secondary reinforcer
   i Token economy
   j Variable ratio reinforcement
   k Variable interval reinforcement

Match the terms above with the descriptions below:

1 Inhibition of unwanted behaviours by association with an unpleasant consequence

2 Receiving a monthly salary

3 Removal of an aversive stimulus increases the probability of the behaviour

4 Produces a high rate of responses, and extinction is slow

4 Classical conditioning:
   a Generalisation
   b Extinction
   c Incubation
   d Stimulus preparedness
   e Discrimination
   f Higher-order conditioning
   g Unconditioned stimulus
   h Conditioned stimulus

Match the terms above with the descriptions below:

   1 Some stimuli are more likely to become conditioned stimuli than others.

   2 The original conditioned stimulus acts as the unconditioned stimulus.

   3 An increase in strength of the conditioned response resulting from repeated brief exposure to the conditioned stimulus.

   4 Gradual disappearance of the conditioned response when the conditioned stimulus is presented without the unconditioned stimulus.

5 Attachment:
   a Indiscriminate attachment
   b Disorganised attachment
   c Discriminate attachment
   d Anxious-avoidant attachment
   e Secure attachment
   f Reciprocal relationship
   g Anxious-resistant relationship
   h Transitional objects
   i Pre-attachment

Select the most appropriate phase or style of attachment for the following situations:

1 The child stays close to the mother and appears anxious even when she is near.

2 The child explores while the mother is in the room and is upset when she leaves.

3 The child ignores the mother and is indifferent to her departure or return.

4 Children are able to have meaningful exchanges with others apart from the main caregiver.

6 Psychosocial development:
a Identity vs. role confusion
b Integrity vs. despair
c Trust vs. mistrust
d Industry vs. inferiority
e Generativity vs. stagnation
f Autonomy vs. shame/doubt
g Intimacy vs. isolation
h Initiative vs. guilt

Select the most appropriate developmental stage for the age ranges below:

1 12–18 years

2 40–65 years

3 3–6 years

7 Moral development:
   a Post-conventional morality
   b Obedience to authority
   c Conventional morality
   d Rewards
   e Individual principles of conscience
   f Pre-conventional morality
   g Good intentions
   h Difference between moral and legal rights
   i Punishment and obedience

Select the most appropriate of Kohlberg's 6 stages and 3 levels (above) for the statements below:

1 The views of others are important, with approval being sought. (3 answers)

2 They are achieved by only 10% of adults. (3 answers)

3 They correspond to Piaget's pre-operational stage. (3 answers)

8 Developmental stages:
   a Concrete operational
   b Oral stage
   c Integrity vs. despair
   d Autonomy vs. shame/doubt
   e Sensorimotor
   f Trust vs. mistrust
   g Anal stage
   h Industry vs. inferiority
   i Latent stage
   j Formal operational
   k Genital stage

Select which developmental stages occur between the following ages:

1   18 months to 3 years (2 answers)

2   7 years to 11 years (3 answers)

3   Birth to 18 months (3 answers)

Answers

MCQs

1   d

The Gestalt principles of perceptual organisation state that we perceive objects not as isolated things but as organised wholes using the laws of closure, continuity, similarity and proximity. (Puri, Hall, p. 11)

2   a

Positive reinforcement occurs in operant conditioning and involves something positive being given to increase the likelihood that the behaviour will reoccur. (Gupta, Gupta, p. 9)

3   c

(Puri, Hall, p. 41)

4   e

Children become proficient as a result of encouragement to speak.

5   d

6   c

Episodic memory is also known as autobiographical memory. (Gupta, Gupta, p. 66)

7   d

Penis envy occurs in girls as they pass from the phallic to the latency stage.

8   d

Festinger described cognitive dissonance as the psychological state that occurs when there is a perceived inconsistency between ideas. It is uncomfortable and motivates the person to reduce dissonance by changing their behaviour or their cognitions. (Gupta, Gupta, p. 137)

9 e

Variable ratio reinforcement is very good at maintaining a high response rate and extinction is slow. (Puri, Hall, p. 6)

10 a

It is the opposite. (Puri, Hall, p. 50)

11 c

This occurs at 12 months. (Puri, Hall, p. 72)

12 b

The Boston Naming Test is a language test. (Puri, Hall, pp. 93–6)

13 a

Life events can have an aetiological role in psychiatric disorders. (Puri, Hall, p. 140)

14 c

15 d

(Puri, Hall, p. 4)

16 c

(Puri, Hall, p. 69)

17 b

18 e

Less than 10% reach the highest level of moral development.

19 a

(Gupta, Gupta, pp. 6–12)

20 a

21 d

(Gross, p. 464)

22 b

Developmental retardation is a long-term effect of privation (i.e. lack/absence of an attachment figure). (Gross, p. 467)

23 c

Amnesia is a memory deficiency, not a theory of forgetting. (Fear, p. 15)

24 a

Shaping is a learning technique based on approximations of behaviour. (Fear, pp. 13–14)

25 e

(Fear, p. 14)

26 a

(Gross, p. 491)

27 e

(Fear, pp. 17–18)

28 b

(Fear, p. 20)

29 e

30 d

(Gross, p. 480)

31 b

(Gupta, Gupta, pp. 403–4)

32 e

Short-term memory duration is up to 30 seconds. (Gupta, Gupta, pp. 61–4)

33 a

(Puri, Hall, p. 75)

34 d

35 a

36 c

(Fear, p. 14)

37 b

Negative reinforcement is associated with operant conditioning. (Puri, Hall, pp. 3–4)

38 d

Sexual conflict occurs in the phallic stage.

39 a

40 a

(Gross, p. 155)

41 c

(Gross, p. 154)

42 d

Higher-order conditioning occurs in classical conditioning.

43 b

This bipolar visual analogue scale is easy to use and has good test-retest reliability.

44 d

(Puri, Hall, p. 72)

45 c

The paranoid-schizoid position was described by Klein. (Fear, p. 515)

46 d

47 b

This begins at 6–8 months.

48 b

Piaget felt that before the age of 7 the child is egocentric, unable to logically reason, and under the sway of the superficial perceived image.

49 c

Imprinting occurs throughout the animal kingdom.

50 a

This is a classification within the Strange Situation experiment.

51 b

Guilt is a common stage in grief reactions to the death of others. (Gross, p. 568)

52 c

Mahler also described the symbiotic phase and the separation-individuation phase.

53 d

54 c

(Gupta, Gupta, p. 97)

EMIs

1 1 a, j

   2 h

   3 k

   4 d

2 1 g

   2 c

   3 b

   4 d

3 1 c

   2 g

   3 d

   4 j

4 1 d

   2 f

   3 c

   4 b

5 1 g

2 e

3 d

4 f

6 1 a

2 e

3 h

7 1 b, c, g

2 a, e, h

3 d, f, i

8 1 d, g

2 a, h, i

3 b, e, f

Psychopathology

Questions

MCQs

1 Which of the following is not a first rank symptom of schizophrenia?
   a Delusional perception
   b Thought broadcast
   c Somatic passivity
   d Thought block
   e Thought insertion

2 Which of the following is not a symptom of catatonia?
   a Echopraxia
   b Circumstantiality
   c Ambitendency
   d Waxy flexibility
   e Mannerisms

3   Which of the following is not true of thought disorder?
    a   Executive dysfunction contributes to formal thought disorder.
    b   Thought disorder is associated with enhanced semantic priming.
    c   Neologisms are a disorder of the pragmatic aspects of speech.
    d   Continuation of thought disorder after resolution of an acute psychotic episode is a strong predictor of poor outcome.
    e   Formal thought disorder is associated with impaired theory of mind.

4   Which of the following is true of autochthonous delusions?
    a   They may occur in epileptic psychosis.
    b   They explain pre-existing hallucinations.
    c   They are a form of secondary delusion.
    d   They are usually ego-dystonic.
    e   They are a first rank symptom of schizophrenia.

5   Which of the following is true of primary delusions?
    a   They indicate a poor prognosis in schizophrenia.
    b   They are diagnostic of schizophrenia.
    c   They are more common in acute than in chronic schizophrenia.
    d   They are characteristically persecutory.
    e   They refer to a systematised set of beliefs.

6   Which of the following is true of morbid jealousy?
    a   It is more common in females.
    b   It is a misidentification phenomenon.
    c   It excludes real marital infidelity by definition.
    d   It is also referred to as de Clérambault syndrome.
    e   It has been described in dementia.

7   Which of the following is false, regarding overvalued ideas?
    a   They occur in anorexia nervosa.
    b   They are usually associated with abnormal personality.

c They tend to run a chronic course unresponsive to treatment.

d They are maintained with less conviction than delusions.

e They are viewed by the patient as senseless.

8 Which of the following are not common contents of obsessional thoughts?

a Dirt and contamination

b Aggressive actions

c Orderliness

d Sex

e Music

9 Which of the following is true regarding dysmorphophobia?

a It can be symptomatic of schizophrenia.

b It is cured by corrective surgery.

c It increases proportionately with the objective degree of deformity.

d It is always based on an overvalued idea.

e It is a phobic disorder.

10 Which of the following is true regarding obsessions?

a Obsessional thoughts can be overvalued ideas.

b They are typically ego-syntonic.

c They are rare in schizophrenia.

d They are typically distressing.

e They are attributed by the patient to external sources.

11 Which of the following is true regarding confabulation?

a It is a characteristic feature of chronic Korsakoff's syndrome.

b It is associated with anterograde amnesia.

c Sufferers will typically know they have a memory problem.

d It occurs in clouded consciousness.

e It contains no elements of true events.

12 Which of the following is the correct description of the type of hallucination?

a Extracampine hallucinations occur when waking from sleep.

b Functional hallucinations serve a specific purpose.

c Reflex hallucinations occur without an associated trigger.

d Hypnopompic hallucinations occur while falling asleep.

e Pseudohallucinations are intangible and located in inner subjective space and lack substantiality.

13 Which of the following is not a term used to describe formal thought disorder?

a Fusion

b Echopraxia

c Substitution

d Derailment

e Drivelling

14 Which of the following is false regarding alexithymia?

a Patients with alexithymia have difficulty in distinguishing between somatic and psychological feelings.

b There is reduced symbolic thinking.

c It does not contribute to masked depression.

d Patients have difficulty describing their emotions.

e Thinking is literal.

15 Which of the following is false relating to hallucinations?

a They are less vivid than real perceptions.

b They are impossible to distinguish from real perceptions in clear consciousness.

c Auditory hallucinations are invariably heard in external space in schizophrenia.

d They can occur in normal people.

e Auditory hallucinations may be associated with sub-vocal muscle movements.

16 Which of the following is false relating to depersonalisation?

    a It is characteristically unpleasant.

    b It is ego-syntonic.

    c It is always associated with a change in mood.

    d It affects the perception of the passage of time.

    e It occurs in healthy people.

17 In relation to thought disorder, which of the following was not described by Bleuler?

    a Loosening of associations

    b Condensation

    c Faulty use of symbols

    d Omission

    e Displacement

18 Which of the following is not an immature defence mechanism?

    a Projection

    b Denial

    c Splitting

    d Introjection

    e Undoing

19 Which of the following is true regarding formal thought disorder?

    a Loosening of associations is pathognomonic of schizophrenia.

    b Confabulation is a disorder of the form of thought.

    c Tangential thinking is the same as circumstantiality.

    d Executive dysfunction contributes to formal thought disorder.

    e Perseveration is the same as verbal stereotypy.

20 Which of the following is true regarding pseudohallucinations?
   a They are usually under voluntary control.
   b They usually indicate the presence of psychosis.
   c They usually occur in the visual modality.
   d They can be present in Ganser's syndrome.
   e They are usually associated with flat affect.

21 Which of the following is false in relation to flight of ideas?
   a It is characteristic of mania.
   b Clang associations are a feature.
   c It characteristically includes Vorbeireden.
   d It may include punning and rhyming.
   e It can be explained by distraction from external stimuli.

22 Which of the following is true regarding primary delusions?
   a They are first rank symptoms of schizophrenia.
   b They indicate a poor prognosis in schizophrenia.
   c They can be derived from auditory hallucinations.
   d They are more common in chronic schizophrenia.
   e They can be preceded by delusional mood.

23 Which of the following is false regarding overvalued ideas?
   a They can dominate a sufferer's life.
   b They are viewed by the patient as senseless.
   c They tend to have a poor prognosis.
   d They are commonly associated with paranoid personality
     disorder.
   e They occur in dysmorphophobia.

24 Which of the following is true of tangentiality?

  a It is characteristic of mania.

  b It is a disorder of the pragmatic aspects of speech.

  c It is the same as circumstantiality.

  d It is pathognomonic of schizophrenia.

  e It is a reliable marker of imminent relapse in schizophrenia.

25 In relation to thought disorder, which of the following was not described by Cameron?

  a Displacement

  b Metonymy

  c Asyndesis

  d Interpenetration

  e Over-inclusive thinking

26 Which of the following is false regarding depersonalisation?

  a It can be experienced by normal people.

  b Perception of time is altered.

  c People around oneself feel unreal.

  d It is associated with unpleasant emotional states.

  e It can involve changes in tactile sensation.

27 Which of the following is not a connection between thoughts as seen in flight of ideas?

  a Chance relationships

  b Clang associations

  c Derailment

  d Distracting stimuli

  e Verbal associations

28 Which of the following is not an example of an abnormal posture or movement?

  a Ambitendency

  b Echopraxia

  c Negativism

  d Waxy flexibility

  e Palilalia

29 Which of the following definitions is incorrect?

  a Derailment: the thought moves on to a subsidiary thought

  b Drivelling: there is a disordered combination of various thoughts

  c Fusion: heterogeneous elements of thought are interwoven with each other

  d Omission: a thought or part of a thought is senselessly omitted

  e Substitution: a major thought is substituted by a subsidiary thought

30 Which of the following is not a disorder of mood?

  a Apathy

  b Alexithymia

  c Irritability

  d Lability

  e Elation

31 Which of the following is not a neurotic defence mechanism?

  a Reaction formation

  b Projective identification

  c Isolation

  d Dissociation

  e Intellectualisation

32 Which of the following definitions are incorrect?

a Alogophobia: fear of pain

b Zoophobia: fear of animals

c Claustrophobia: fear of closed spaces

d Xenophobia: fear of men

e Acrophobia: fear of heights

33 Which of the following is not a movement disorder?

a Akinesia

b Chorea

c Astereognosia

d Athetosis

e Ambitendency

34 Which of the following is not classically associated with schizophrenia?

a Ambitendency

b Negativism

c Preservation

d Stupor

e Lability

35 Which of the following descriptions is incorrect?

a Confabulation: gaps in memory are unconsciously filled with false memories

b Déjà pense: the illusion of recognition of a false thought

c Jamais vu: the illusion of failure to recognise a familiar situation

d Retrospective falsification: false details are added to the recollection of an otherwise real memory

e Déjà vu: the feeling that the current situation has never happened before

36 Which of the following is not an illusion?

a Micropsia

b Derealisation

c Macropsia

d Misinterpretation

e Pareidolia

37 Which of the following is not a mature defence mechanism?

a Repression

b Sublimation

c Humour

d Suppression

e Altruism

38 Which of the following is true regarding delusions?

a They are reality for the patient.

b They are frequently held by other people.

c They are usually bizarre in nature.

d They are held with a certainty that may be shakeable.

e They always stem from an abnormal perception.

39 In relation to thought disorder, which of the following was not described by Schneider?

a Derailment

b Fusion

c Concrete thinking

d Omission

e Drivelling

40 Which of the following is true?
  a Stereotypies are goal-directed repetitive movements.
  b Chorea consists of slow, writhing movements.
  c Mannerisms are non-goal-directed repetitive movements.
  d Athetosis consists of random, jerky movements.
  e Negativism can be regarded as an accentuation of opposition.

41 Which of the following is true of concrete thinking?
  a It is diagnostic of schizophrenia.
  b It is diagnostic of organic brain disease.
  c It may occur in manic psychosis.
  d It is a defect of conceptual abstract thought.
  e It is tested by asking patients to memorise a list.

42 Which of the following is false in relation to formication?
  a It is a tactile hallucination.
  b It may be seen in delirium.
  c It may be associated with delusions of infestation.
  d It may be seen in psychosis caused by cocaine.
  e It is a passivity phenomenon.

43 A delusional belief that the sexual partner is being unfaithful is known as:
  a Capgras syndrome
  b Othello syndrome
  c Fregoli syndrome
  d Monosymptomatic hypochondriacal psychosis
  e De Clérambault syndrome

44 Which of the following is not a normal experience?

   a Jamais vu

   b Derealisation

   c Delusional perception

   d Hypnagogic hallucinations

   e Depersonalisation

45 Which of the following is true regarding pseudohallucinations?

   a They are subject to conscious manipulation.

   b They are dependent on environmental stimuli.

   c They arise in inner space.

   d They may occur in the real world.

   e They possess the vivid quality of normal perceptions.

46 Which of the following is true regarding obsessive rituals?

   a They respond well to behaviour therapy.

   b They are usually antisocial.

   c They are regarded as sensible.

   d They are not resisted.

   e They reduce anxiety.

47 In which circumstances or people do pseudohallucinations not occur?

   a Dreams

   b Lone prisoners

   c Long-distance lorry drivers

   d Day-dreaming

   e Sensory deprivation

48 Which of the following statements is true?

   a Functional hallucinations are rare in chronic schizophrenia.

   b Autoscopy is synonymous with phantom mirror-image.

   c Reflex hallucinations occur outside sensory field limits.

d In extracampine hallucinations a stimulus in one sensory modality produces a hallucination in another.

e In reflex hallucinations a stimulus in one sensory modality produces a hallucination in the same sensory modality.

49 Which of the following is not a cause of stupor?

a Mania

b Hysteria

c Schizophrenia

d Depression

e Epilepsy

50 Which of the following is true about the first rank symptoms of schizophrenia?

a They incorporate passivity phenomena.

b They are pathognomonic of schizophrenia.

c They only occur in schizophrenia.

d They include formal thought disorder.

e They include incongruity of affect.

51 Which of the following is not a specific feature of catatonic schizophrenia?

a Waxy flexibility

b Palilalia

c Logoclonia

d Tardive dyskinesia

e Psychological pillow

52 Which of the following does not occur in depressive psychosis?

a Delusions of guilt

b Primary delusions

c Delusions of poverty

d Auditory hallucinations

e Cotard's syndrome

53 Which of the following is true regarding erotomania?
   a It is a misidentification syndrome.
   b It can be a feature of obsessive-compulsive disorder.
   c It is seen in Cotard's syndrome.
   d It is also called Othello syndrome.
   e It may result in stalking behaviour.

54 Which of the following is true regarding obsessional thoughts?
   a They always give rise to compulsions.
   b They are ego-dystonic.
   c They are rarely of a sexual nature.
   d They usually respond to imipramine.
   e They do not occur in schizophrenia.

55 Which of the following is true about elementary hallucinations?
   a They can occur in the form of thought echoes.
   b They can be flashes of light.
   c They can be audible thoughts.
   d They can include hearing voices.
   e They can include seeing animals.

56 Which of the following is not a movement disorder?
   a Stereotypy
   b Athetosis
   c Ambitendency
   d Mitmachen
   e Verbigeration

57 Which of the following is not a formal thought disorder?
   a Gegenhalten
   b Verbigeration
   c Loosening of associations
   d Vorbeireden
   e Knight's move

58 Which of the following is not a speech or language disorder?

  a Alogia

  b Alexia

  c Apophany

  d Coprolalia

  e Neologism

59 Which of the following is not a property of defence mechanisms?

  a They are unconscious.

  b They help manage instincts and affects.

  c There are seven basic types.

  d They are dynamic and reversible.

  e They are mostly adaptive.

EMIs

1 Disorders of perception:

  a Completion illusion

  b Functional hallucination

  c Pareidolic illusion

  d Extracampine hallucination

  e Reflex hallucination

  f Affect illusion

  g Hypnagogic hallucination

  h Hypnopompic hallucination

  i Synaesthesia

Which of the above disorders of perception are described below?

  1 A patient hears voices alongside the broadcast voices when the television or radio is on.

  2 When a patient hears running water she feels her flesh is being torn from her body.

3 A man hears the shopkeeper in the next town talking about him.

4 A man who has been recently widowed sees his dead wife in the garden.

2 Psychiatric syndromes:
 a Capgras syndrome
 b Charles-Bonnet syndrome
 c Cotard's syndrome
 d Couvade syndrome
 e De Clérambault syndrome
 f Ekbom's syndrome
 g Fregoli syndrome
 h Othello syndrome

The following descriptions exemplify which of the above syndromes?

1 A man believes his wife has been replaced by an exact double.

2 A man complains of food cravings, nausea and abdominal pain and is preoccupied with his wife's pregnancy.

3 A young woman believes Robbie Williams is in love with her, and despite the fact that he does not reply to any of her letters she waits outside his house for him.

4 A patient believes that various people she meets are her neighbour in different disguises.

3 Defence mechanisms:
 a Splitting
 b Projective identification
 c Denial
 d Sublimation
 e Repression

f   Reaction formation

g   Displacement

h   Regression

i   Introjection

j   Intellectualisation

k   Suppression

l   Altruism

How can the defence mechanisms above be categorised?

1   Mature defences (3 answers)

2   Immature defences (5 answers)

3   Neurotic defences (4 answers)

4   Delusions:
   a   Nihilistic delusion
   b   Delusional mood
   c   Somatic passivity
   d   Grandiose delusion
   e   Secondary delusion
   f   Delusion of reference
   g   Delusional perception
   h   Delusional memory

Which type of delusion is described below?

1   A 20-year-old man is troubled by the feeling that something unusual is going on and things are not the way they should be.

2   A 39-year-old woman, whose mental illness has lasted for 4 years, claims that her health had been affected since she had an operation at the age of 18 to implant a secret listening device in her stomach.

3 A 42-year-old man is watching television and sees a story about a girl who has been abducted and is convinced that the government are trying to tell him that they will kidnap him.

4 A 25-year-old woman, who has felt for some time that something ominous is going to happen, sees a man in the street talking on a mobile phone and is sure this means that al-Qaeda are plotting to kill her.

5 Disorders of thought and language:
a Neologisms
b Concrete thinking
c Fusion
d Asyndesis
e Paragrammatism
f Tangentiality
g Substitution
h Metonymy
i Condensation
j Derailment

Which of the above terms is described below?

1 Blending two ideas into a false concept

2 Heterogeneous elements of the thought are interwoven

3 Imprecise approximations instead of a more exact word

6 Passivity phenomena:
a Thought withdrawal
b Thought insertion
c Thought broadcast
d Passivity of affect
e Passivity of impulse

f Passivity of volition

g Somatic passivity

Which of these passivity phenomena are exemplified below?

1 'Thoughts are beamed into my mind by a satellite.'

2 'I am a puppet who is manipulated by cosmic strings; when the strings are pulled my body moves and I can't prevent it.'

3 'The chip in my head means that my thoughts are transmitted to everyone.'

7 Motor disorders:
   a Mannerism
   b Chorea
   c Stereotypy
   d Dystonia
   e Tics
   f Hemiballism
   g Akathisia
   h Tardive dyskinesia
   i Catalepsy

Which of the above motor disorders are described in the scenarios below?

1 A woman's husband complains that she keeps pulling odd faces and sticking her tongue out. She has been on depot antipsychotic medication for many years.

2 A man with a long history of schizophrenia repeatedly stands up and salutes for no reason.

3 A young man on the ward complains of painful neck stiffness three days after being prescribed haloperidol.

4   A man on long-term antipsychotic treatment complains of rest-lessness and is constantly tapping his feet on the floor.

8   Disorders of perception:
   a   Palinopsia
   b   Functional hallucination
   c   Pareidolic illusion
   d   Extracampine hallucination
   e   Reflex hallucination
   f   Affect illusion
   g   Hypnagogic hallucination
   h   Hypnopompic hallucination
   i   Synaesthesia

Which disorders of perception are described in the scenarios below?

1   A woman sees the traces of objects as they move around.

2   A man hears the colour red.

3   A child wakes in the night and sees a burglar hiding in the shadows.

4   A woman sees the face of her father in the clouds.

9   Catatonia:
   a   Waxy flexibility
   b   Automatism
   c   Mannerisms
   d   Stereotypies
   e   Ambitendency
   f   Mitgehen
   g   Negativism
   h   Posturing

Which signs of catatonia are described below?

1 Repetitive, goal-directed movements

2 Alternating cooperation and opposition

3 Maintenance of unusual postures for long periods of time against gravity or resistance

10 Defences:
   a Splitting
   b Projective identification
   c Denial
   d Sublimation
   e Repression
   f Reaction formation
   g Displacement
   h Regression
   i Introjection
   j Intellectualisation
   k Suppression
   l Altruism

Which of these defences are described below?

1 Described by Klein (2 answers)

2 Transforming a disturbing idea into its opposite

3 Directing a forbidden impulse towards a socially acceptable end

4 Consciously deciding to postpone paying attention to an impulse or conflict

5 Redirecting feelings from their original object to a more acceptable substitute

Answers

MCQs

1 d

Thought block is not a first rank symptom of schizophrenia, as it is difficult to distinguish it from some form or retardation or other difficulty with thinking. (Sims, p. 165)

2 b

3 c

A neologism is a new word that is created to fill a semantic gap. (Sims, p. 182)

4 a

Autochthonous delusions arise suddenly 'out of the blue' and are a type of primary delusion. (Sims, p. 123)

5 c

6 e

Morbid jealousy is also referred to as Othello syndrome and can occur in all the major psychiatric disorders. It is more common in men and can be highly dangerous. (Casey, Kelly, p. 125)

7 e

An overvalued idea is an acceptable, comprehensible idea pursued by the patient beyond the bounds of reason. (Sims, pp. 143–4)

8 e

9 a

10 d

One of the most important features of obsessions is that their content is often of a nature that causes the sufferer great anxiety. (Casey, Kelly, pp. 36–7)

11 b

Confabulation is more common in the early stages of Korsakoff's syndrome. It is the falsification of memory occurring in clear consciousness in association with organic pathology. (Sims, p. 60)

12 e

(Casey, Kelly, pp. 26–8)

13 b

Echopraxia is the automatic imitation by one person of another person's movements. (Puri, Hall, p. 148)

14 c

(Sims, pp. 309–10)

15 a

16 b

(Casey, Kelly, pp. 75–7)

17 d

Omission was described by Schneider.

18 e

Undoing is a neurotic defence mechanism.

19 d

20 d

(Casey, Kelly, pp. 18–19)

21 c

Vorbeireden is talking past the point, and it occurs in schizophrenia and Ganser's syndrome. (Casey, Kelly, p. 49)

22 e

(Casey, Kelly, pp. 39–40)

23 b

24 b

25 a

Displacement was described by Bleuler.

26 c

This is derealisation.

27 c

This is an example of formal thought disorder

28 e

Palilalia is a form of speech perseveration. (Puri, Hall, p. 149)

29 b

In drivelling there is a disordered intermixture of the constituent parts of one complex thought rather than various thoughts. (Puri, Hall, p. 150)

30 d

Lability is a disorder of affect. (Puri, Hall, p. 150)

31 b

Projective identification is an immature defence mechanism.

32 d

Xenophobia is a fear of strangers. (Puri, Hall, p. 152)

33 c

Astereognosia is the disorder whereby objects cannot be recognised by palpation.

34 e

Lability is commonly seen in mania, personality disorder and organic disorders – especially brainstem lesions.

35 e

Déjà vu is the feeling that the current situation has happened before. (Puri, Hall, p. 155)

36 d

37 a

Repression is a neurotic defence mechanism.

38 a

39 c

Concrete thinking was described by Goldstein.

40 e

Mannerisms are goal directed and stereotypies are not. (Casey, Kelly, pp. 91–6)

41 d

(Sims, pp. 158–9)

42 e

(Casey, Kelly, p. 24)

43 b

44 c

Delusional perception is a first rank symptom of schizophrenia. (Sims, p. 164)

45 c

46 e

47 a

48 b

(Casey, Kelly, pp. 26–7)

49 b

Stupor is a state of more or less complete loss of activity where there is no reaction to external stimuli. (Casey, Kelly, pp. 100–1)

50 a

(Sims, p. 164)

51 d

Tardive dyskinesia may be present in patients presenting for the first time with schizophrenia but is not a specific feature of catatonic schizophrenia. (Casey, Kelly, p. 93)

52 b

Delusions would be secondary to the mood disorder.

53 e

Erotomania is also called de Clérambault syndrome. Othello syndrome is also referred to as morbid jealousy. (Casey, Kelly, pp. 123–5)

54 b

55 b

56 e

Verbigeration is a thought disorder and is also known as 'word salad'.

57 a

Gegenhalten is where patients oppose attempts at passive movement.

58 c

Apophany is a primary delusional experience as described by Conrad, 1958. (Fear, p. 106)

59 c

There are many more than 7 types.

EMIs

1 1   b

2   e

3   d

4   f

2 1   a

2   d

3   e

4   g

3 1   d, k, l

2   a, b, c, h, i

3   e, f, g, j

4 1 b

   2 h

   3 f

   4 g

5 1 i

   2 c

   3 h

6 1 b

   2 f

   3 c

7 1 h

   2 a

   3 d

   4 g

8 1 a

   2 i

   3 f

   4 c

9 1 c

   2 e

3   a

10 1   a, b

2   f

3   d

4   k

5   g

6

Aetiology and prevention

Questions

MCQs

1 Which of the following is an example of primary prevention?
   a Education about substance misuse
   b Outreach support
   c Assessment of carer needs
   d Rehabilitation services for patients with schizophrenia
   e Adherence compliance programmes

2 How many life years are lost through suicide amongst males in the UK?
   a 10000
   b 20000
   c 50000
   d 75000
   e 100000

3 What percentage of people will experience some kind of mental health problem over the course of a year?
   a 5%
   b 10%
   c 15%
   d 20%
   e 25%

4 Which of the following is not a risk factor for completed suicide?

a Male gender

b Young age

c Depressive illness

d Family history

e Alcohol

5 Which of the following is not an example of a suicide reduction strategy?

a Restricting paracetamol availability

b Signs with the Samaritans' contact details displayed on high bridges

c Shotgun licence restrictions

d Health and safety checks on psychiatric inpatient units

e Compulsory catalytic converters on motor vehicles

6 What term refers to those strategies that are aimed to minimise handicap if recovery is not complete?

a Primary prevention

b Secondary prevention

c Tertiary prevention

d Public health intervention

e Reintegration

7 What is the approximate concordance rate for schizophrenia in monozygotic twins?

a 45%

b 5%

c 20%

d 65%

e 10%

8 Which of the following is true regarding suicide in England and Wales?

    a It occurs at similar age-specific rates to those in Scotland.

    b It is commoner in unskilled social classes than in professional social classes.

    c It is more common in women.

    d It is predominantly a problem of young to middle life.

    e It occurs more frequently in the spring and summer.

9 What is a person's risk of schizophrenia if both parents have schizophrenia?

    a 5%

    b 15%

    c 25%

    d 45%

    e 60%

10 Which of the following is a dynamic risk factor?

    a Previous violence

    b Male gender

    c History of substance misuse

    d Previous poor compliance with treatment

    e Command hallucinations

11 Which of the following is a risk factor for schizophrenia?

    a Childhood sexual abuse

    b Reduced visual acuity

    c Smoking

    d Impaired hearing

    e Perinatal hypoxia

12 Which of the following statements is false regarding prognosis in bipolar affective disorder?

   a The long-term outcome is worse than for unipolar depression.

   b 90% of patients with mania experience further episodes.

   c The interval between episodes increases with increasing age and number of episodes.

   d Rapid-cycling disorders have a poorer prognosis.

   e Bipolar II disorders have a better prognosis than bipolar I disorders.

13 Which of the following statements about alcohol dependence is true?

   a There is equal monozygotic and dizygotic concordance for alcoholism.

   b There is a two-fold increase in the risk of alcoholism in first-degree relatives.

   c There are higher rates of conduct disorder in sons of alcoholic parents.

   d Sons of alcoholics are more likely to become alcoholics if raised by their biological parents than if adopted.

   e A co-morbid psychiatric diagnosis is uncommon.

14 Which of the following is a risk factor for depression?

   a Loss of mother before the age of 14 years

   b Regular use of NSAIDs

   c Being a migrant

   d Being an oldest child

   e Childhood sexual abuse

15 Which of the following statements about the neurobiological basis of schizophrenia is false?

   a Enlarged lateral ventricles correlate with poor clinical outcome.

   b Negative symptomatology can be mimicked by phencyclidine.

c Drug-naive patients with schizophrenia have increased D2 receptor density compared to controls.

d Decreased cortical volume and enlarged ventricles are present at first presentation.

e Drug-free patients with schizophrenia show elevated dopamine release in response to an amphetamine challenge in comparison to controls.

16 Which of the following is not one of Beck's cognitive distortions in depression?

a Selective abstraction

b Systematic desensitisation

c Overgeneralisation

d Arbitrary inference

e Worthlessness

17 Which of the following factors is associated with good prognosis in schizophrenia?

a Negative symptoms

b Precipitating event

c Insidious onset

d Poor concordance with medication

e Poor social network

18 Which of the following statements about bipolar affective disorder is true?

a It never occurs for the first time after the age of 65.

b The risk of bipolar disorder in first-degree relatives is 15%.

c There is no increased risk of unipolar depression in first-degree relatives.

d The mean age of onset is earlier than for unipolar depression.

e It is more common in females.

19 Which of the following statements about schizophrenia is false?

   a There is an increased risk in those with learning disability.

   b The risk of schizophrenia is increased by 5 times in first-degree relatives.

   c Urban birth increases the incidence.

   d Two affected parents confer a 46% risk that the child will have schizophrenia.

   e An increased risk is associated with Huntingdon's chorea.

20 Which of the following statements about the neurobiological basis of depression is false?

   a Decreased 5HIAA levels in the CSF have been described.

   b Trytophan availability is increased in depression.

   c Basal cortisol levels are elevated in acutely depressed patients.

   d Blunted 5HT mediated prolactin release has been described.

   e Free T3 levels may be decreased.

21 Which of the following statements about anorexia nervosa is correct?

   a Premature birth is an independent risk factor.

   b It is strongly correlated with shoplifting.

   c Concordance rates are similar for monozygotic and dizygotic twins.

   d It is overrepresented in lower social classes.

   e It is not more common in enmeshed families.

22 Which of the following may be a maintaining factor in the aetiology of schizophrenia?

   a Family history of schizophrenia

   b Parental separation/loss

   c Childhood abuse

   d High expressed emotion

   e Birth complications

23 Which of the following statements is true regarding suicide risk?

   a Multiple-suicide attempters show no differences in presence of childhood abuse when compared with single-suicide attempters.

   b There is no evidence for a genetic contribution in suicide that aggregates in families.

   c Suicides are more likely during the week than at weekends.

   d Social taboo concerning suicide is not shown to impact on suicide rate.

   e Patients with dissocial personality disorder have an increased risk of completed suicide after presenting with deliberate self-harm.

24 What is the approximate prevalence rate of unipolar depression in first-degree relatives of those with unipolar affective disorders?

   a 0–5%

   b 5–10%

   c 10–15%

   d 15–20%

   e 20–25%

25 Which of the following is not a risk factor for very late onset schizophrenia?

   a Female gender

   b Hearing impairment

   c Living alone

   d Visual impairment

   e Schizophrenia in first-degree relatives

26 Which of the following is not a psychological theory of depression?

a Maternal deprivation

b Learned helplessness

c Klein – failure of the child to pass through the 'depressive position'

d Freud – regression to the anal stage of psychosexual development

e Freud – regression to the oral stage of psychosexual development

EMIs

1 Aetiology:

a Female gender

b Unemployment

c Visual impairment

d Living alone

e Male gender

f Recent discharge from hospital

g Low IQ

h Being married

i Past psychiatric history

Select three of the above which are risk factors for:

1 Suicide (3 answers)

2 Depression (3 answers)

3 Late onset schizophrenia (3 answers)

Answers

MCQs

1 a

Primary prevention is a population-based strategy aimed at modifying the risk factors for a given disorder. (Fear, p. 280)

2 e

Men's Health Forum, 2006. (menshealthforum.org.uk)

3 e

Goldberg D. Filters to care. In: Jenkins R, Griffiths S, editors. *Indicators for Mental Health in the Population*. London: The Stationery Office; 1991.

4 b

The elderly are at increased risk of completed suicide.

5 e

This has reduced suicides, but via an incidental route.

6 c

(Fear, p. 281)

7 a

It is 10% in dizygotic twins.

8 e

Monthly rates rise by approximately 10% in the spring and summer.

9 d

10 e

The other options are all static (historical) risk factors.

11 e

12 c

The interval between episodes decreases with increasing age and number of episodes.

13 c

There is a 7-fold increase in alcoholism in first-degree relatives. Being adopted does not alter the risk of alcoholism in the sons of alcoholics.

14 a

As reported by Brown and Harris in 1978. (Puri, Hall, p. 140–1)

15 a

16 e

(Gross, p. 650)

17 b

18 d

The risk of bipolar disorder in first-degree relatives is 8%.

19 b

The risk is increased 10-fold in first-degree relatives.

20 b

It is reduced.

21 a

22 d

The remaining options are all predisposing factors.

23 e

24 c

25 e

There is no increased risk of schizophrenia in first-degree relatives in very late onset schizophrenia.

26 d

This is a psychoanalytical theory for obsessional symptoms.

EMIs

1 1   b, e, f

2   a, d, i

3   a, c, d

History, ethics and philosophy, stigma and culture

Questions

MCQs

1   In which year did Bleuler first use the term 'schizophrenia'?
    a   1881
    b   1891
    c   1901
    d   1911
    e   1921

2   Which of the following ethical principles refers to the patient's right to choose their treatment?
    a   Non-maleficence
    b   Beneficence
    c   Autonomy
    d   Justice
    e   Confidentiality

3 Which of the following is a Royal College of Psychiatrists anti-stigma campaign?

a Reduce

b Changing Minds

c Partners in Care

d SHIFT

e See Me

4 Which of the following ethical principles indicates that all patients should be treated equally?

a Non-maleficence

b Beneficence

c Autonomy

d Justice

e Confidentiality

5 What percentage of people with mental health problems have experienced harassment while living in communities?

a 20–25%

b 30–35%

c 40–45%

d 50–55%

e 60–65%

6 What percentage of people on incapacity benefit have a mental illness?

a 10%

b 20%

c 30%

d 40%

e 50%

7 Regarding confidentiality, which of the following is not true?

a Children over the age of 16 should enjoy the same rights of confidentiality as adults.

b Without consent, information cannot be shared with relatives, even in the patient's best interests.

c Effective measures should be taken to protect personal information.

d Disclosure of information should be kept to a minimum and consent should be obtained.

e Wherever possible, unidentifiable information should be used.

8 In the assessment of capacity to give consent, which of the following is not relevant?

a Patient's ability to comprehend the relevant information

b Patient's ability to trust their doctor

c Patient's ability to communicate their decision

d Patient's ability to retain the relevant information for sufficient time

e Patient's ability to believe the information

9 Which of the following ethnic groups consumes the most alcohol?

a British Muslims

b Hindus

c White British

d Afro-Caribbeans in the UK

e Blacks in the USA

10 Which of the following is not associated with the anti-psychiatry movement?

a Ladislas J Meduna

b Erving Goffman

c Michel Foucault

d Thomas Szasz

e RD Laing

11 In which decade did John Cade discover the benefits of using lithium in mania?

a 1900s

b 1910s

c 1920s

d 1930s

e 1940s

12 People from which ethnic group seek help about psychiatric symptoms the least?

a White British

b Black British

c British Asian

d British Chinese

e Mixed Ethnicity

13 In which year was chlorpromazine's effectiveness in treating schizophrenia discovered?

a 1932

b 1942

c 1952

d 1962

e 1972

14 Regarding the Declaration of Geneva, which of the following is false?

a It includes a statement about respecting medical teachers.

b It includes guidance on confidentiality.

c It refers to colleagues as sisters and brothers.

d It was intended as a revision of the Oath of Hippocrates.

e It is not relevant in modern day medicine.

15 Which of the following is false about culture-bound syndromes?

a Koro is fear that the penis is shrinking into the abdomen.

b Piblokto occurs among Eskimos.

c Windigo is a manic condition.

d Amok is associated with South-East Asia.

e Susto is anxiety related to loss of the soul.

16 Which of the following is true about the history of schizophrenia?

a Kraepelin introduced the term 'schizophrenia'.

b Bleuler's primary symptoms for diagnosis included anhedonia.

c Jaspers believed that the essential feature of the schizophrenic experience is that it is not understandable.

d Bleuler coined the term 'dementia praecox'.

e Schneider held that first rank symptoms were essential for the diagnosis.

17 Which of the following cultural-bound syndromes is an anxiety associated with fear of the penis retracting into the abdomen, resulting in death?

a Koro

b Amok

c Latah

d Dhat

e Susto

18 Which body of beliefs is opposed to psychiatry?

a Meher Baba

b Wahhabism

c Missionaries of Charity

d Church of Scientology

e The Essenes

19 Which best describes the medical ethical principle of non-maleficence?

   a First, do no harm.

   b Act in the best interest of the patient.

   c The patient must be treated with dignity.

   d All patients must be treated equally.

   e The patient has the right to choose their treatment.

20 Which of the following terms is not associated with Emil Kraepelin?

   a Dementia praecox

   b Schizophrenia

   c Manic-depression

   d Alzheimer's disease

   e Paedophilia

21 Which of the following is false about the history of bipolar affective disorder?

   a Genetic studies suggest that bipolar and unipolar depression may lie along a spectrum.

   b Kraepelin made a distinction between dementia praecox and manic-depressive psychosis.

   c There has been no subsequent evidence to challenge the Kraepelinian dichotomy.

   d Leonhard made a distinction between bipolar and monopolar depression.

   e Bleuler viewed dementia praecox and manic-depressive psychosis as occurring along a continuum.

22 Which of the following is not one of Bleuler's fundamental symptoms of schizophrenia?

a Autism

b Ambivalence

c Incongruity of affect

d Loosening of association

e Auditory hallucinations

23 In which year was Erving Goffman's book *Stigma: notes on the management of spoiled identity* published?

a 1933

b 1943

c 1953

d 1963

e 1973

24 Which of the following is incorrect in relation to historical theories of the aetiology of schizophrenia?

a A schizophrenogenic mother is both overprotective and hostile towards her children.

b Double bind was a concept described by Bateman.

c Marital skew is when one parent yields to the eccentric wishes of the other dominant parent.

d The schizophrenogenic mother was described by Lidz.

e Double bind involves incongruent messages being the prevalent mode of communication with the child.

25 Which of the following is false about culture-bound syndromes?

a Koro is an acute anxiety state.

b Latah is an hysterical reaction to stress.

c Windigo is a depressive psychosis.

d Amok is an acute anxiety state.

e Dhat is a psychosexual disorder.

EMIs

1 Culture-bound syndromes:
   a Brain fag
   b Amok
   c Dhat
   d Latah
   e Pibloko
   f Susto
   g Koro
   h Windigo

Select which of the above syndromes fits with the following descriptions:

1 A fear that the genitals are retracting into the abdomen

2 A West African student complains of reduced concentration, poor memory and neck pain

3 An acute dissociative state occurring in Eskimo women

4 A belief that semen is being lost in the urine causing exhaustion

Answers

MCQs

1 d

2 c

3 b

SHIFT (National Institute for Mental Health in England) and See Me (alliance of Scottish mental health organisations) are also anti-stigma campaigns (*see* rcpsych.ac.uk for further details).

4 d

5 c

41% according to the Scottish NSF (2001).

6 d

Sainsbury Centre for Mental Health. *The Economic and Social Costs of Mental Illness.* London: SCMH; 2003.

7 b

In special circumstances (e.g. dementia), information can be shared when the patient is unable to give consent and it is in their best interests.

8 b

9 c

Kessler RC, McGonagle KA, Zhao S *et al.* Lifetime and 12-month prevalence of DSM-III-R psychiatric disorders in the United States. Results from the National Comorbidity Survey. *Arch Gen Psychiatry.* 1994; **51**(1): 8–19.

10 a

Ladislas J Meduna introduced ECT in 1934.

11 e

John Cade was an Australian psychiatrist.

12 c

(Murray J, Williams P. Self-reported illness and general practice consultations in Asian-born and British-born residents of West London. *Soc Psychiatry*. 1986; **21**(3): 136–145. Gillam SJ, Jarman B, White P *et al*. Ethnic differences in consultation rates in urban general practice. *BMJ*. 1989; **299**: 953–957.)

13 c

14 e

The Declaration of Geneva has been adopted by the World Medical Association and was last updated in 2006.

15 c

Windigo is a depressive condition with the delusion that one has become cannibalistic. (Casey, Kelly, pp. 122–3)

16 c

17 a

Koro is a culture-bound syndrome that is found in Malaysia and South China and best understood as an acute anxiety state.

18 d

The Church of Scientology was established in 1952 and has a strong following among celebrities in Los Angeles.

19 a

This is a one of the core values that apply to medical ethics.

20 b

Kraepelin distinguished between manic-depression and dementia praecox, which was later named schizophrenia (Kraepelin never used the term). Kraepelin also co-discovered Alzheimer's disease and spent much of his time researching paedophilia.

21 c

Recent genetic studies indicate that bipolar affective disorder, schizo-affective disorder and schizophrenia may lie on a continuum.

22 e

Bleuler's '4 As' of schizophrenia are: Autism, loosening of Associations, Ambivalence, incongruity of Affect.

23 d

In this book Goffman sought to analyse 3 types of stigma.

24 d

Lidz described martial skew and schism. The schizophrenogenic mother was described by Fromm-Reichmann.

25 d

Amok is a depressive or dissociative disorder associated with South-East Asia. (Casey, Kelly, pp. 122–3)

EMIs

1 1 g

   2 a

   3 e

   4 c

Index

Key: (Q) = question, (A) = answer

The New MRCPsych Paper I Practice MCQs and EMIs